Earth Day
Edible Earth Goes
Soccer Ball

Whole Foods Signature

Michele Jeanmarie

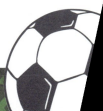

Archway Publishing books may be ordered through booksellers or by contacting:

Archway Publishing
1663 Liberty Drive
Bloomington, IN 47403
www.archwaypublishing.com
844-669-3957

Interior Image Credit: Aaron Herrera

ISBN: 978-1-6657-6191-8 (sc)
ISBN: 978-1-6657-6192-5 (e)

Print information available on the last page.

Archway Publishing rev. date: 06/20/2024

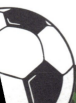
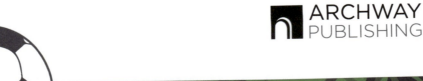

Earth Day
Edible Earth Goes
Soccer Ball

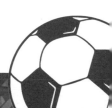

It was now past midafternoon. The sun was still blustering. All day soccer ball was sitting on the lawn, lonely, abandoned, neglected. Everyone was coming in and out, going and coming, coming and going. Cars were passing by. School buses were rolling. Soccer ball was all alone.

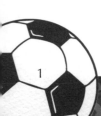

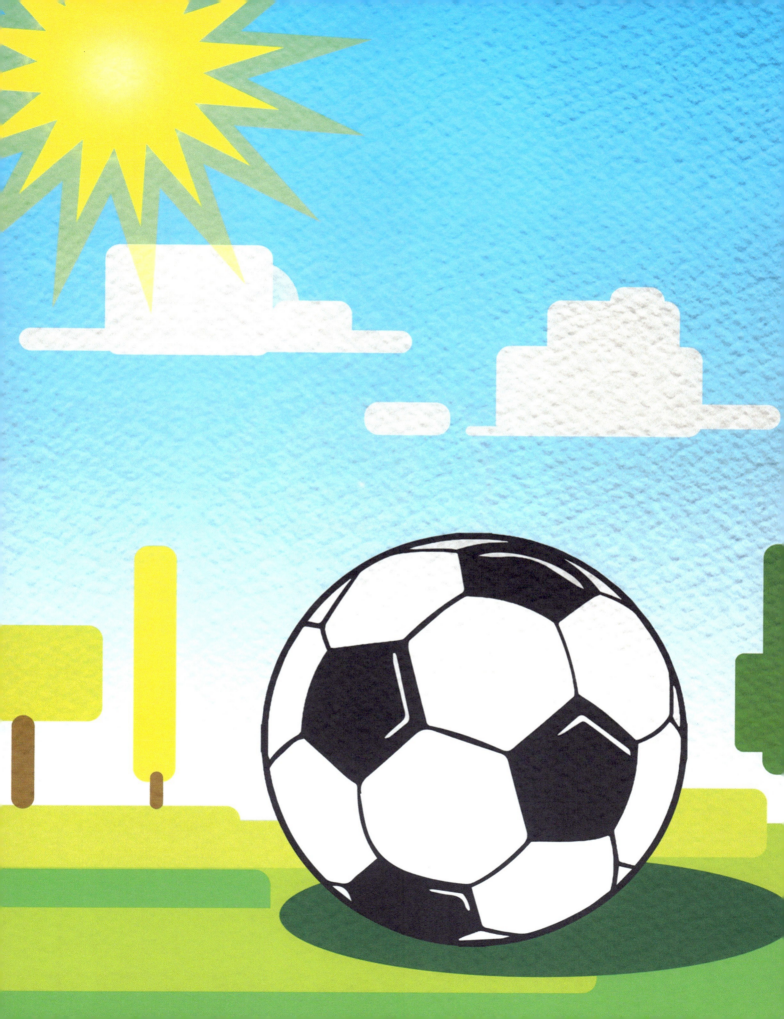

Suddenly, soccer ball hears screeching. Children were finally coming home. All of a sudden, soccer ball felt a ballistic kick. BOOM!

"Whew, I am alive," shouted soccer ball, "yippee! If ever I were so glad to be kicked over here. I must now wander."

"What a beautiful garden," thinks soccer ball. "Beautiful garden, beautiful me. I shall now be called, César, the soccer ball."

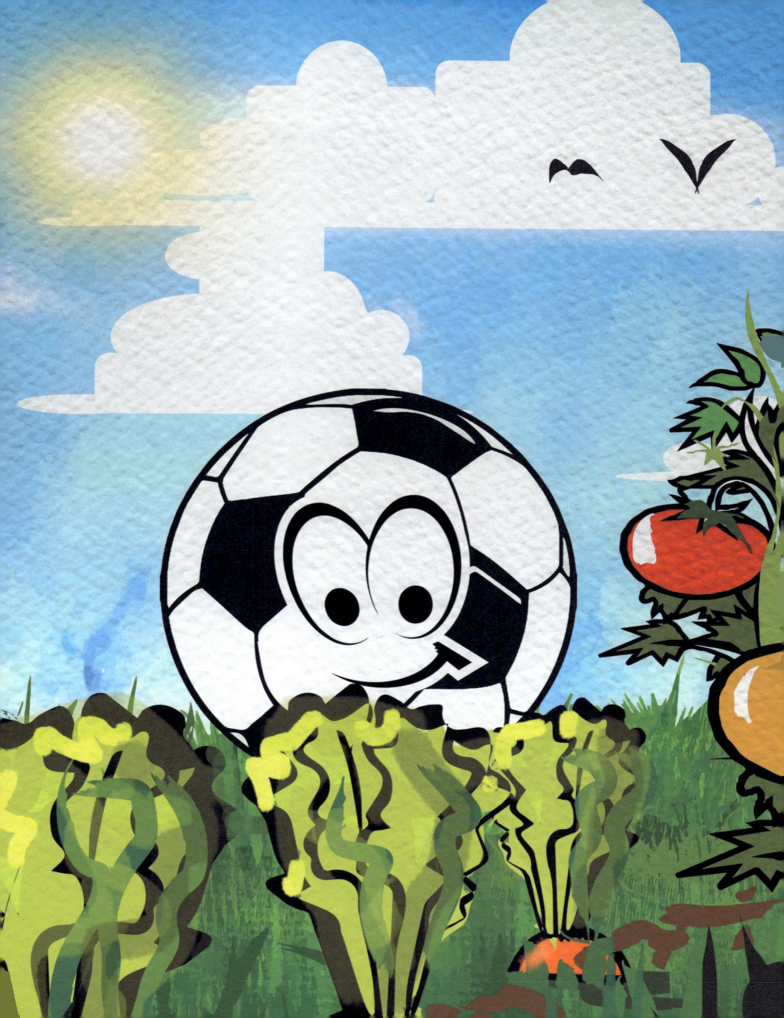

Rolling along, César, the soccer ball comes across a patch of green skinny leaves. "They sure look different." He yanks a patch, and up springs carrot.

"Hey!" moans carrot.

César, the soccer ball leaps backward and slices it. "Scrunch, scrunch," he goes.

Then silence.

"What do I do with these?" Thinks César, the soccer ball. He yanks up another slice.

"Wait! Before you go ballistic, I am good for you," whispers carrot.

"Ballistic," he interrupts. "I did become César, the soccer ball, because someone went BALL-IS-TIC on me!"

He pauses, "now, tell me; how are you good for me?" César, the soccer ball asks.

"Well, see my concentric circles?" carrot points. "See the little circle; see the middle circle; see the larger circle? They are like your eyes, and that makes me good for your eyesight.

"I see," agrees César, the soccer ball, and swipes up two slices before he goes, "there!"

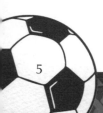

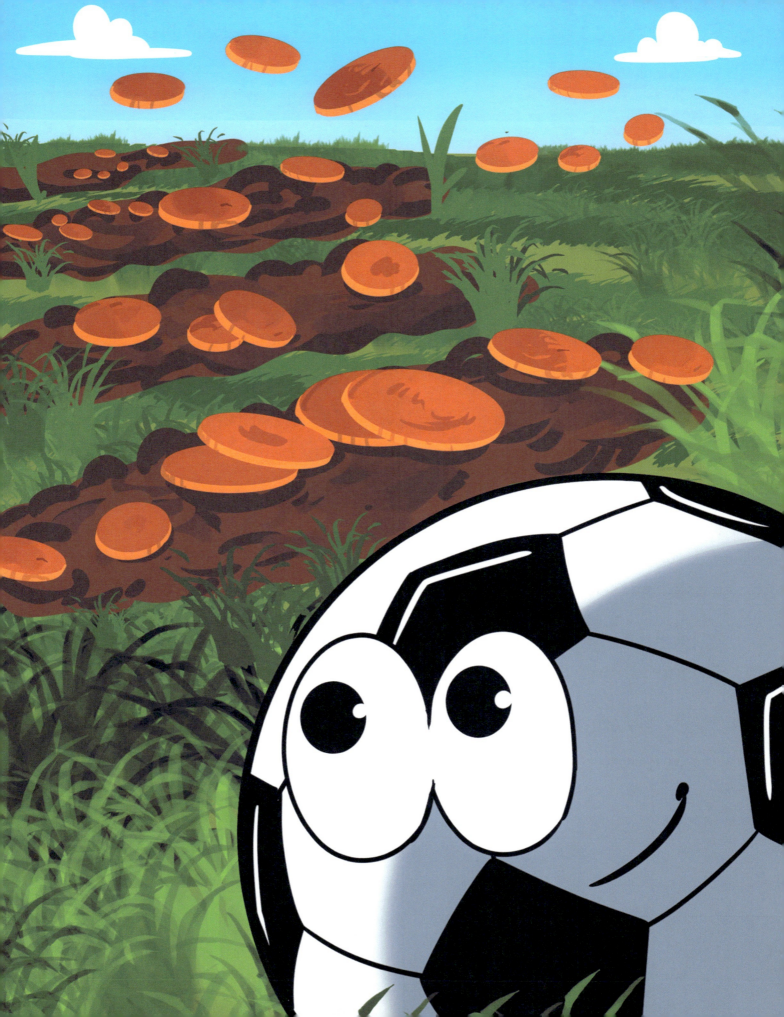

"Boing, boing," goes César, the soccer ball, until red tomato comes a-rolling-forth!

"Forth and back, back and forth," thought César, the soccer ball. So, he rolls himself towards it and splits it open.

"Hmm! What did I do?" asks César, the soccer ball. "Eat your tomato!" demands a voice. César, the soccer ball rolls back.

"Who speaks?"

"Do you not see the four sections? Each section is called a chamber." César, the soccer ball turns to tomato.

"The heart has four chambers, and like the tomato, it is also red. Science shows that tomatoes are food for the blood."

"So..., eat your tomatoes," he hears again. He swoops one up and, "Down they go!"

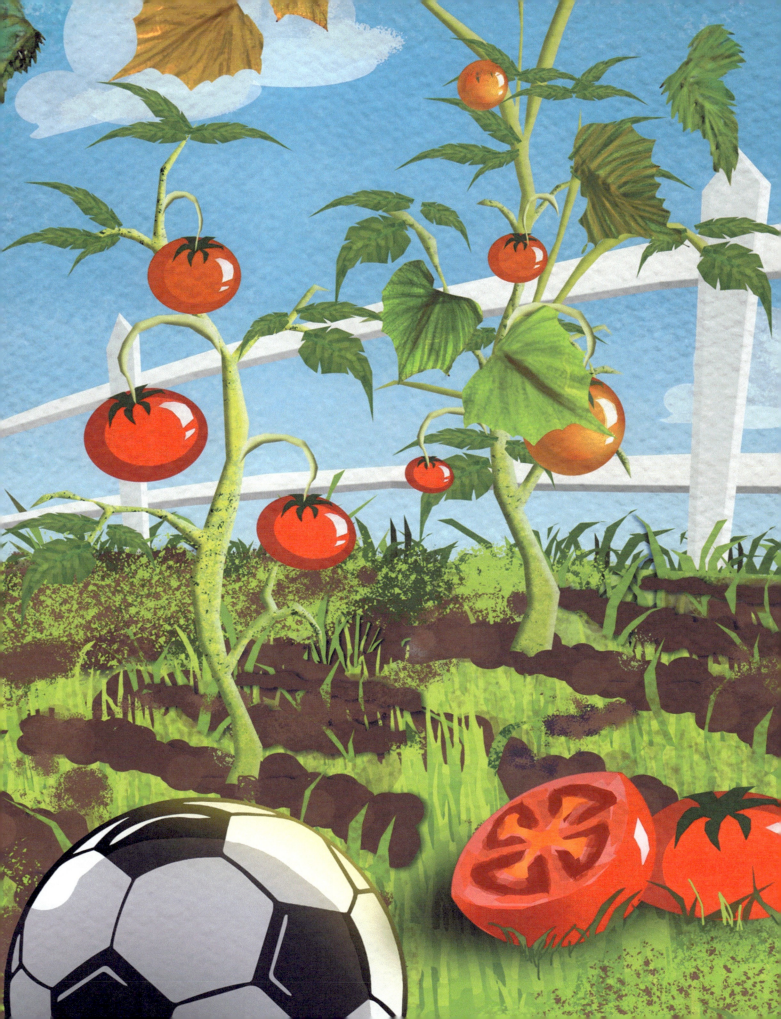

"Boing, boing," goes César, the soccer ball, until grapes, in the wind, swing back and forth, but oh-oh! They are tangled.

"What are you?" Thinks César, the soccer ball. "What good are you for?"

"I am all sewed up," so César, the soccer ball unsews a cluster.

"Look at me, just one of us," order grapes. "Doesn't one of us look like a blood cell? They have been using us to make drinks. They pluck us. They stomp on us. They dance on us. They put us into barrels. They leave us there for a long time, then they drink us." Grapes add, "do you see us hanging in clusters? Aren't we shaped like a heart?"

César, the soccer ball looks on and ponders, "so, grapes are food for the heart, you say."

César, the soccer ball picks up a cluster of grapes. "Down they go!"

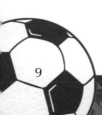

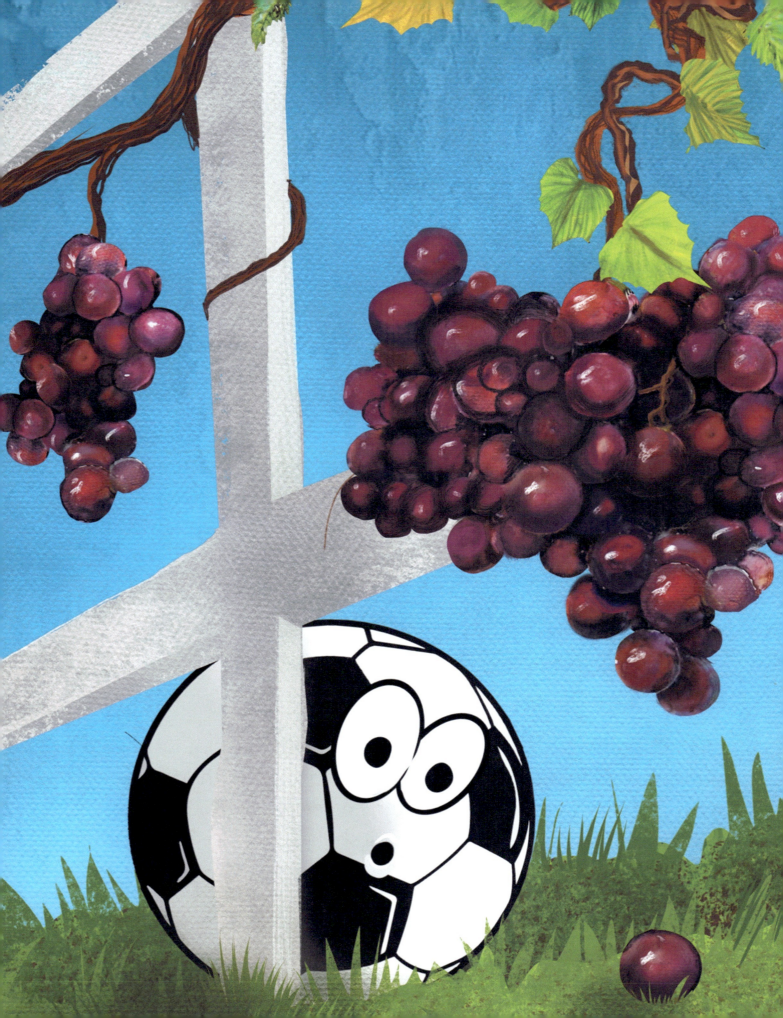

"Boing, boing," goes César, the soccer ball when from a tree, walnut goes, "plops!"

César, the soccer ball shouts. "The sky is falling," but then sees what hit him on the head was a walnut.

"Howdy," salutes walnut.

Curiosity gets the best of him. César, the soccer ball stomps and cracks open the walnut when he hears exclaimed, "The brain! The brain! There are two halves of us, like the brain. Each side is called a hemisphere."

"See," walnut adds, "There is a left hemisphere and a right hemisphere. Each hemisphere has an upper section and a lower section."

Walnut continues, "The upper section is called cerebrum, and the lower section is called the cerebellum."

Walnut reproaches, "The thing you stepped on is called a case. Like the case that protects your brain, we have a case that protects us, too!"

"See the wrinkles?" walnut stares. "The wrinkles are just like the ones on your brain. They are like little highways that connect to each other. When you learn something new, a new highway opens. When you don't use your highway, it shuts down. So, keep learning to keep those highways improving."

"Wow, I better take one, then." César, the soccer ball nestles it down.

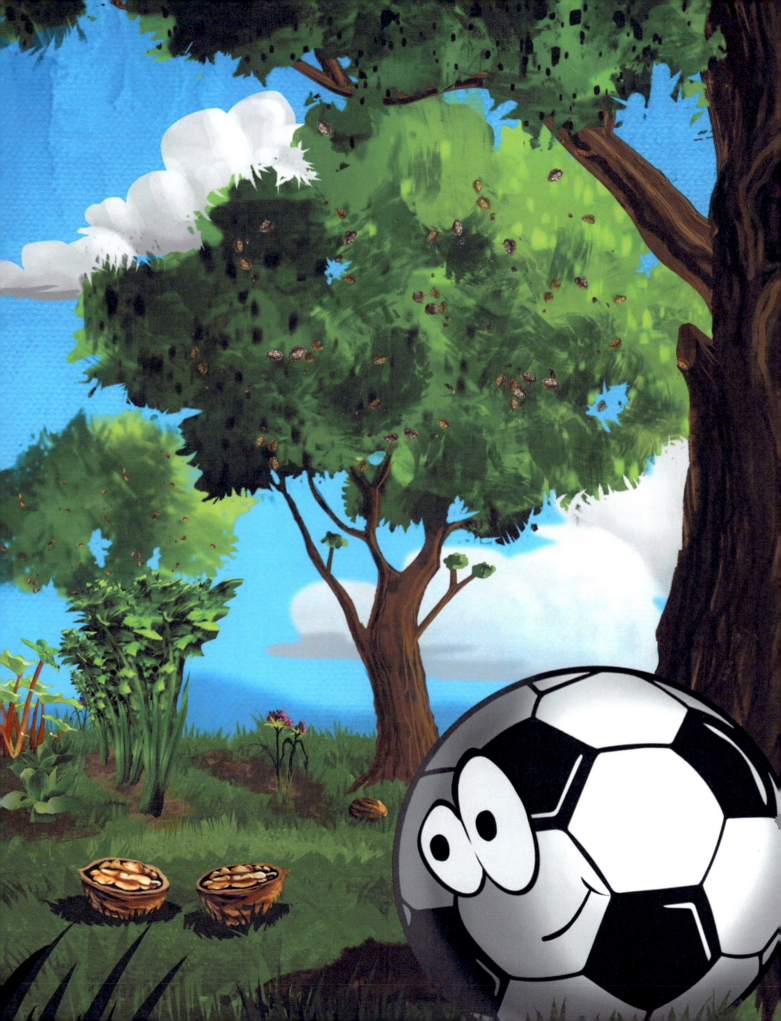

"Boing, boing," goes César, the soccer ball, landing in a stalk of kidney beans. Kidney bean goes, "what's kicking?

"Nothing's kicking?" responds César, the soccer ball. César, the soccer ball picks up two pods and looks at them.

"That's the kidney. Kidney beans help the kidney function. We balance the acids in your bodies. Acids include orange juice, grapefruit juice, cranberry juice and lemonade.

We remove wastes from your bodies, too, those that hurt your tummies.

We control your blood pressure. When you run for the school bus, and you are breathing hard, and you get hot, you have a need to cool down, right? Well, we balance those extremes, too.

We also convert vitamin D, so when you drink milk and eat cheese and yogurt, the milk and cheese and yogurt are converted to make you stronger.

We even balance the water in your bodies. We produce something in your bodies that makes more red blood cells."

"Do you remember the fruit that helps the blood?" asks kidney. "Grapes!" exclaims a voice. César, the soccer ball peeks around, but nothing. "Down they go!"

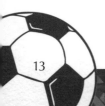

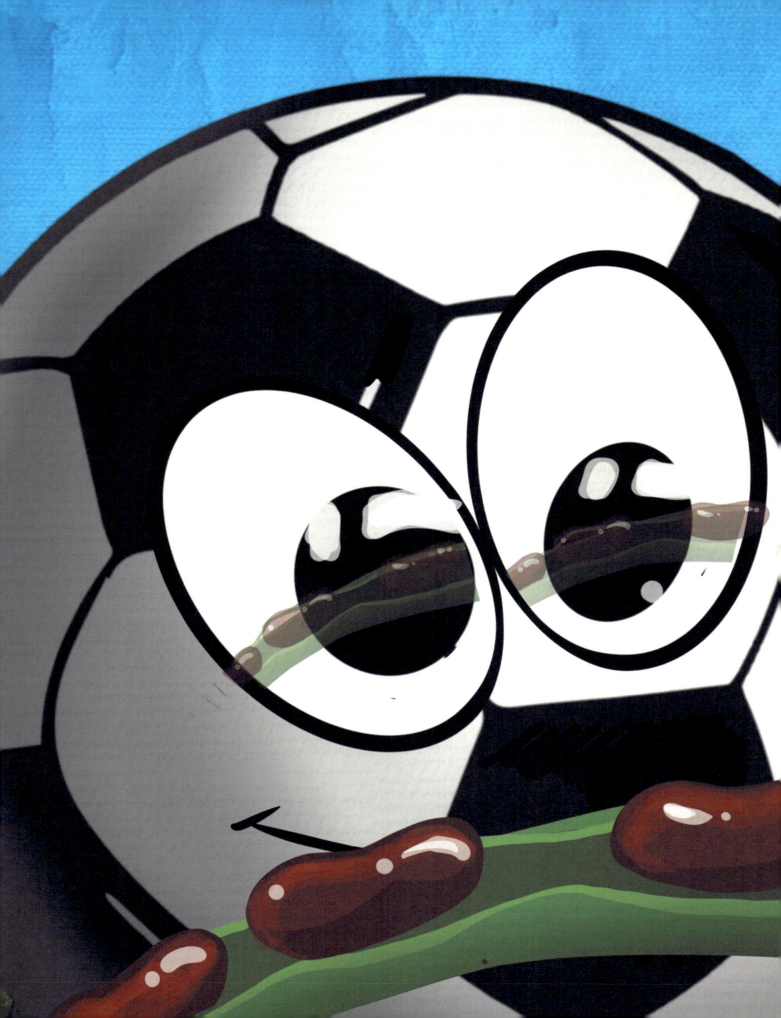

"Boing, boing," goes César, the soccer ball, until celery, bok choy, and rhubarb did the kicking!"

"I am pooped," slumps César, the soccer ball. "I need a pick-me-up."

"You have come to the right place," celery, bok choy, and rhubarb concede.

"How so?" asks César, the soccer ball.

He snaps one stalk and closely observes. Celery, bok choy, and rhubarb, and others like it look just like bones.

"Hey, can you strengthen my legs?" "We sure can!"

"Eat these. We strengthen bones. Bones are made up of 23% salt, and..., these foods are also 23% salt. If you don't eat enough of these, your body will pull it from other bones in your body, making them weak."

César, the soccer ball settles on quite a few. "Down they go!"

"How many bones are in the human body?" ponder celery, bok choy, and rhubarb.

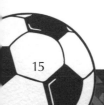

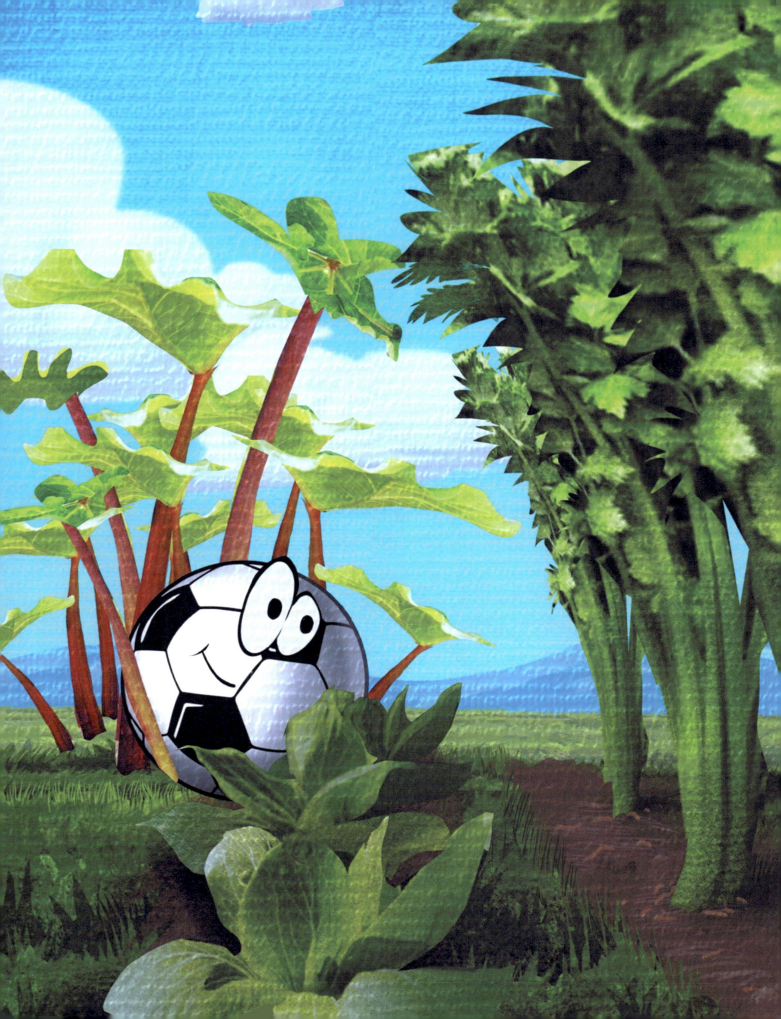

"Boing, boing," goes César, the soccer ball, until figs go, "Newton." "What are you?" Thinks César, the soccer ball.

César, the soccer ball slices the fig when suddenly, figs go berserk. He spits out a bunch of itsy, bitsy, tiny seeds at him. Figs hang and grow in twos. They swim about the body, as if it is nobody's business.

"Who is there?" I heard some giggling. César, the soccer ball decides on two. "Down they go!"

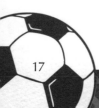

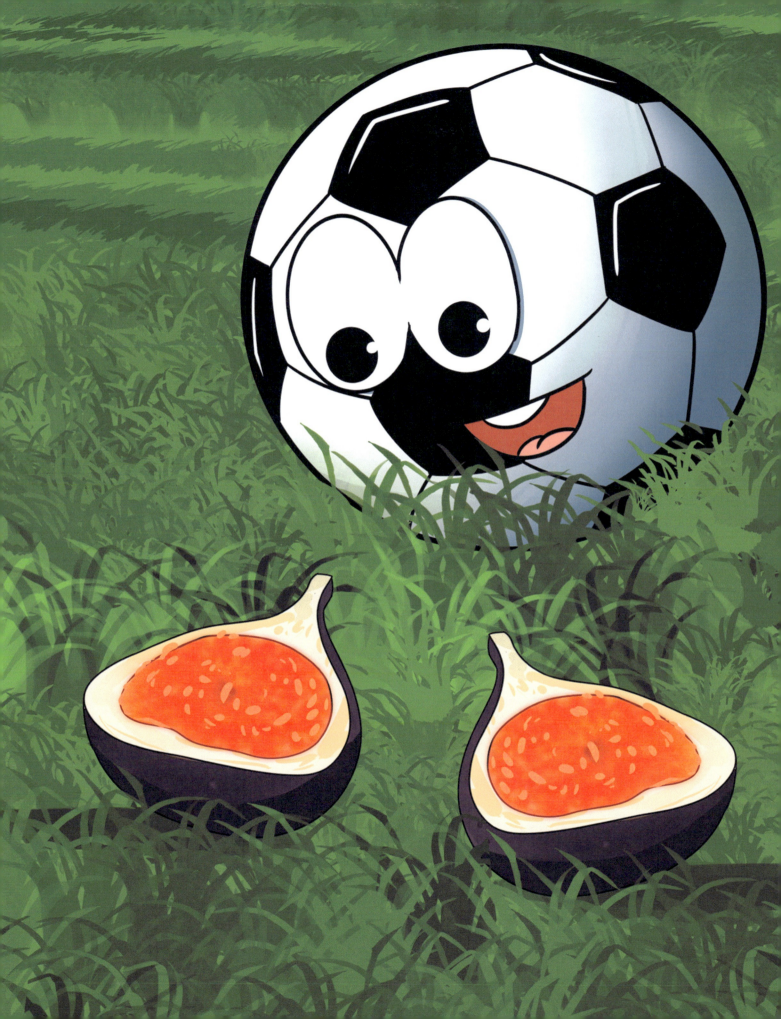

"Boing, boing," goes César, the soccer ball, until eggplant, avocadoes, and pears go, "squish!"

"Who are you?" they ask.

"I am César, the soccer ball. Speak up. Tell me about yourselves!"

César, the soccer ball tilts one way, then another way.

Eggplant, avocadoes and pears reply, "we keep mommies' tummies healthy until babies are ready to leave."

"Huh?"

"Eating avocado puts one in a better mood. So, when you are feeling down, EAT an avocado," shouts eggplant of avocado.

"Another thing," It also sheds baby weight and prevents bad cells from forming in mommies' tummies," clarify pears.

"Won't you know, it takes exactly nine months to grow an avocado from flower to fruit?" boasts eggplant of avocado. "Do you know what else takes nine months to grow?"

"Babies," hears César, the soccer ball. He swerves around, but sees nothing, so he plucks one of each. "Down they go!"

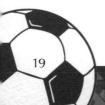

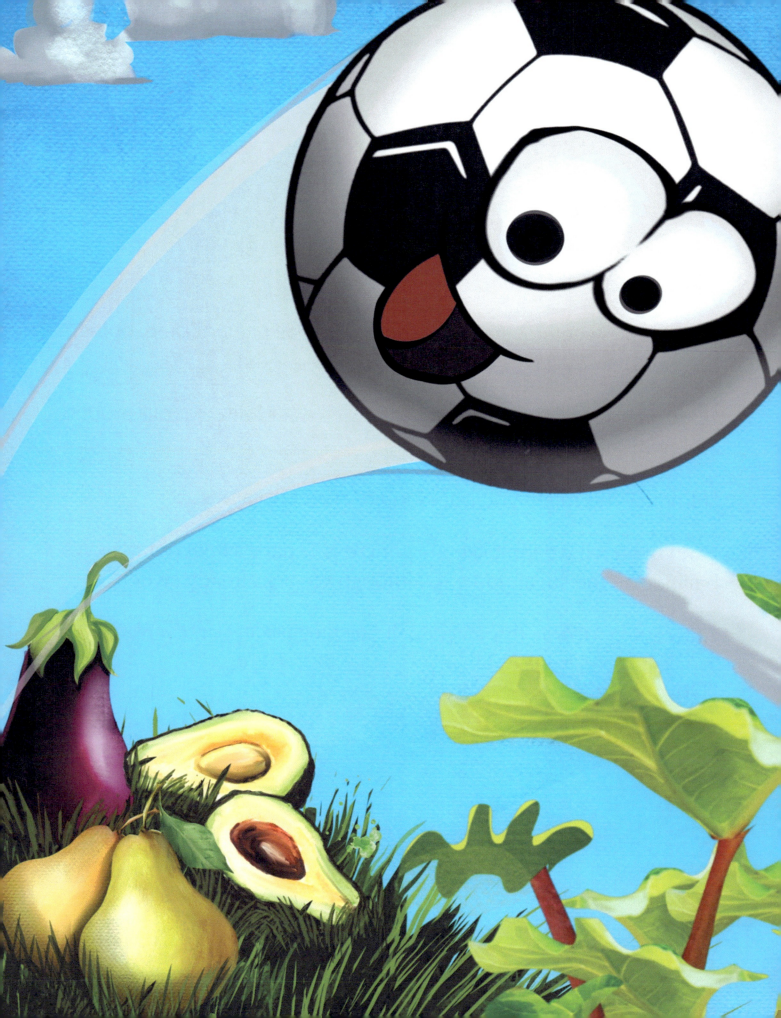

Up Mount Sweet Potato César, the soccer ball goes, "Boing, boing," he goes until SWEET POTATOES go, "s-w-e-e-et!"

"Explain yourself," demands César, the soccer ball. He rolls around and twirls around.

"Hmm...Who might you be?" inquire sweet potatoes.

"Can't you tell we look like the pancreas," snarls sweet potato. "We balance all the sugar you eat, although we are already sweet."

"Interesting," César, the soccer ball puzzlingly states and yanks three.

"Down they go!"

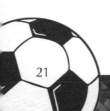

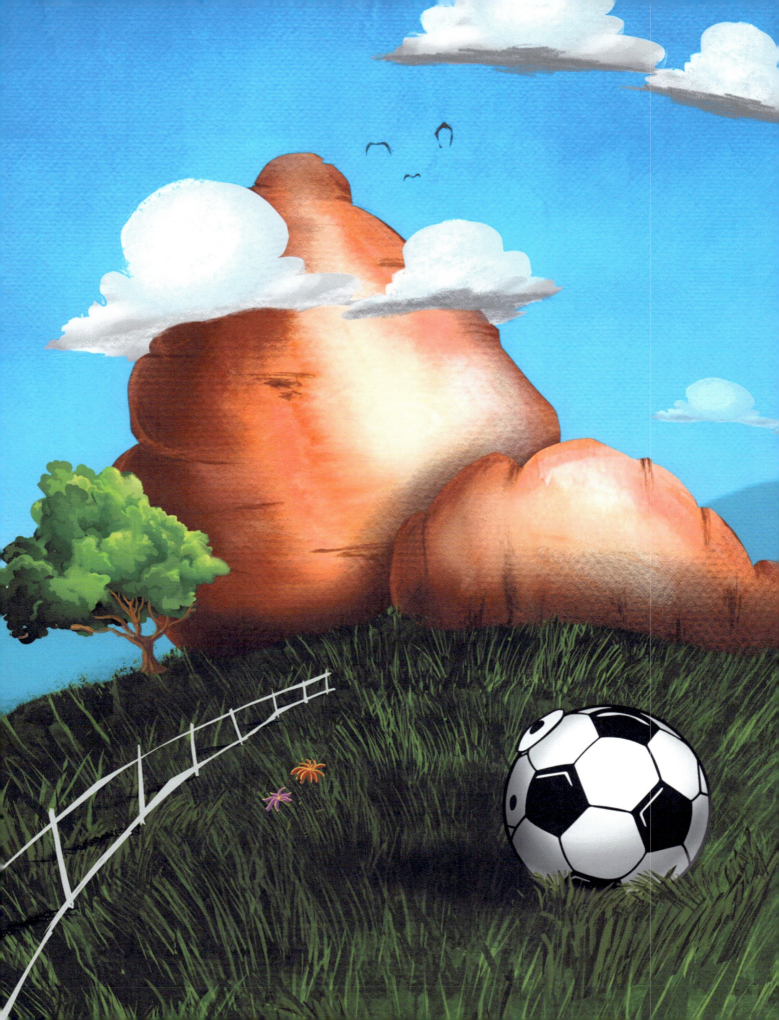

"Boing, boing," goes César, the soccer ball, until olives go, "olé!" "And you?" César, the soccer ball asks.

"We are ovals," they reply. "What in your body are ovals?"

"Ovaries!"

"That's right! We are part of the Mediterranean diet. Some of our trees have been around for over a thousand years. Aren't we something?" they brag.

César, the soccer ball collects two. "Down they go!"

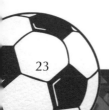

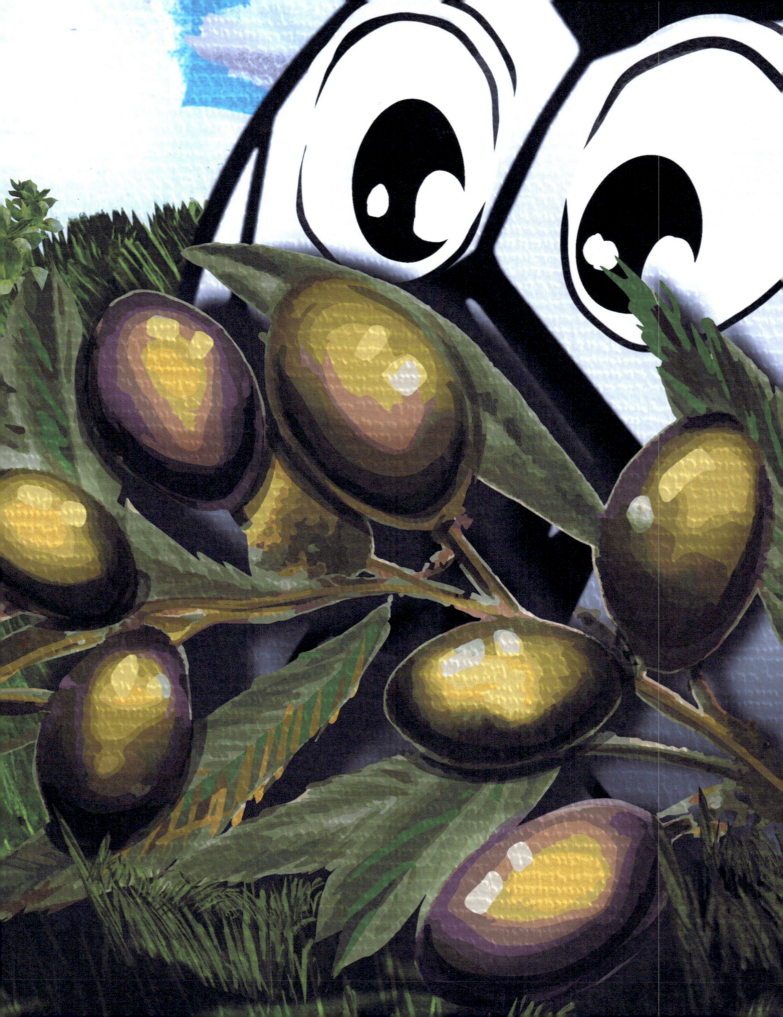

"Boing, boing," goes César, the soccer ball, until grapefruits, oranges, and citrus fruits go, "peel!"

"Speak!" commands César, the soccer ball. "I see you are round, like me," perceives César, the soccer ball.

Grapefruits, oranges and citrus fruits look just like those to which babies cling for milk. Milk, very important. César, the soccer ball twists off two.

"Down they go!"

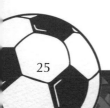

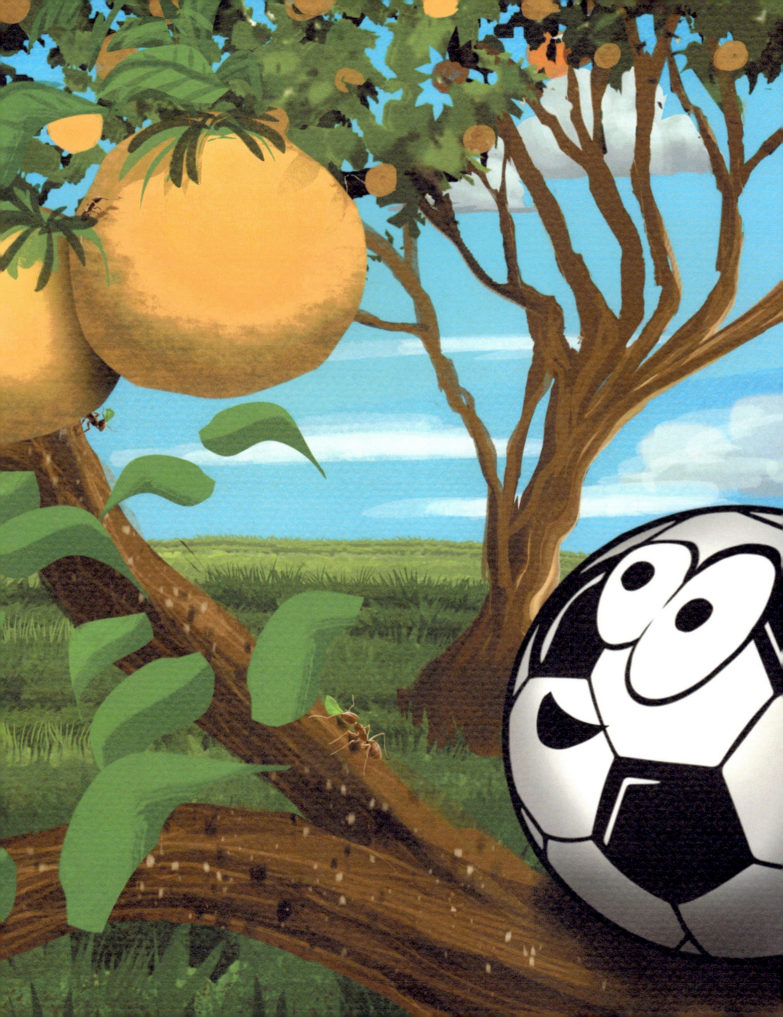

"Boing, boing," goes César, the soccer ball, until onions go "teary!" "I am getting tired," admits César, the soccer ball.

"How can these help?" thinks César, the soccer ball. He gets closer. He smells. He slices. He squints and bats his eyes.

Onions look just like the skin.

"We block things from entering the onion, so when things enter your body through the eyes, the nose, and the mouth, the onion helps the body rid itself of them."

César, the soccer ball opts for a few. "Down they go!"

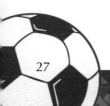

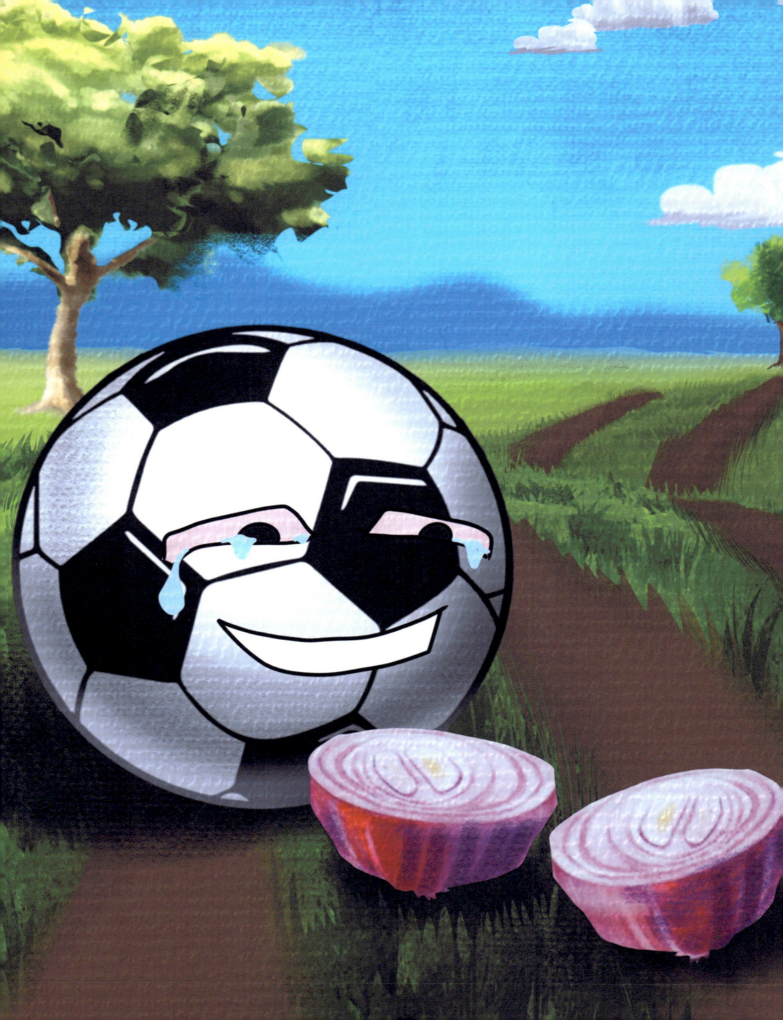

Another rustle.

Not bothering, César, the soccer ball takes a final look. "Look at what I just sculpted?"

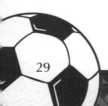

Draw an outline of your anatomy. Place each Whole Foods Signature in its appropriate place.

Then comes a voice, "Earth Day, Edible Earth. Eat vegetables! Eat fruits."

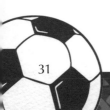

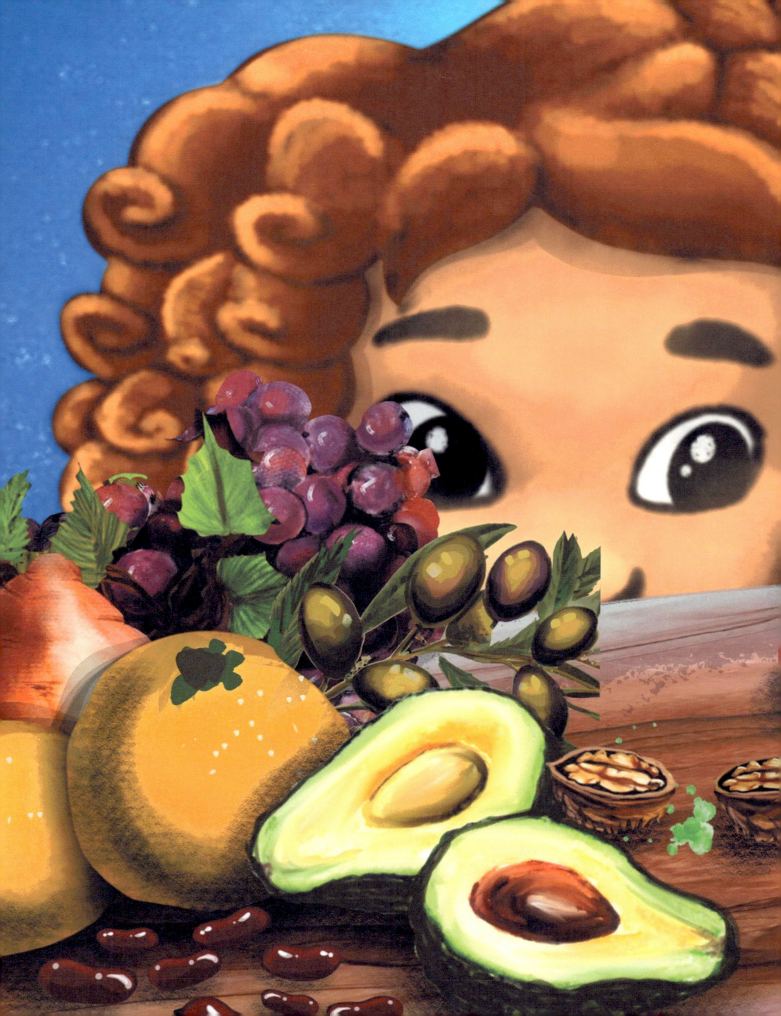

ACTIVITIES ACROSS THE DISCIPLINES

Also Known As:
Integrated Studies

It is known also as interdisciplinary studies.

It involves several topics and themes across disciplines to promote and engage student readers throughout the study.

It aims to target different learning styles offering multiple avenues to guide comprehension.

It is an effective approach in helping students become multifaceted learners while developing expertise in the discipline of choice.

It is a network of disciplines that enable students to develop meaningful understanding of complex associations.

It is coupled with project-based learning that makes school more interesting and productive for students and teachers alike.

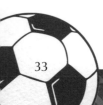

EARTH DAY, EDIBLE EARTH GOES SOCCER BALL

A Matching Game For Older Kids

Match:

1. Sperm	_____ a. Olive
2. Heart	_____ b. Sweet potato
3. Kidney	_____ c. Figs
4. Brain	_____ d. Grapefruit
5. Eyes	_____ e. Onion
6. Bones	_____ f. Celery/Rhubarb/Bok choy
7. Breasts	_____ g. Walnut
8. Ovaries	_____ h. Tomato
9. Blood Cells	_____ i. Carrot
10. Pancreas	_____ j. Bean
11. Cervix/ Womb	_____ k. Grapes
12. Skin	_____ l. Avocado/Eggplant/Pear

How many are attributed to the reproductive system?

EARTH DAY EDIBLE
EARTH GOES SOCCER BALL

Science and Art Integration:

Materials:
Roll of butcher paper, or wrapping paper, or newspaper
Scissors
Glue
Magazines
Real or plastic fruits and vegetables mentioned in the story
(feel free to sketch them, cut and glue)

Directions:
Pair up.
Roll out the butcher paper. Outline each other's full body, at least, to the thighs.
Read, "Earth Day Edible Earth Goes Soccer Ball."
Find photos of the fruits and vegetables mentioned in the story.
Cut them out.
Alternatively, sketch them.
Alternatively, pick up some plastic versions from the craft store.
Alternatively, use the real fruits and vegetables, in which case, you will need special glue to adhere them to the butcher paper cut-out. You will also need shellac or inexpensive hair spray to spray them down to keep the critters away.
Take a picture. Post on your favorite platform.

Hashtag#EarthDayEdibleEarthGoesSoccerBall
Hashtag#MicheleJeanmarie
Hashtag#ChelasBooksandThings

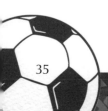

Rubric

Did pairs work in harmony?

10 points

Did you trace out and cut out the body neatly?

25 points

Did you cut out and glued the fruits and vegetables neatly?

25 points

Did you include all 12 fruits?

25 points

Free

15 points

Total

EARTH DAY EDiBLE
EARTH GOES SOCCER BALL

I. Technology Integration:

Create a TikTok challenge. Use one or two fruits and vegetables from the story. In a cooking demonstration, create or duplicate a quick recipe. Add music. Dance while you create it. Challenge your followers to another video.

Hashtag#EarthDayEdibleEarthGoesSoccerBall
Hashtag#MicheleJeanmarie
Hashtag#ChelasBooksandThings

Have fun!

YouTube Challenge
YouTube Big Dill Maya Rudolph + Seventh Generation.

II. Grammar Integration:

Define a homophones.
List the homophones the actor used.

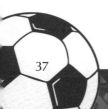

EARTH DAY EDIBLE
EARTH GOES SOCCER BALL

Theology Integration:

Unlike popular belief, the fig tree was in the middle of the garden. It was the forbidden fruit, yet Lucifer coaxed Eve, who coaxed Adam to take from it. They both ate the fig. Lucifer was made to crawl on his belly, becoming the nemesis of man. Eve and all women were to labor in pain. Adam and all men were to work from sunup to sundown. From being able to enjoy freely from the garden, both Adam and Eve, our first parents, are relegated to work.

Is that statement still true? How so?

Explain from earth we came, to earth we shall return.

What came first: creation of the garden or Adam? Cite your source. Copy it here:

Who was given the task of naming each food and animal? Cite your source. Copy it here:

The fruits and vegetables mentioned in this story are known as WHOLE FOODS SIGNATURE.

Why would they be known as signature? Whose signature could it be?
The fig, the avocado, the pear, the eggplant, the grapefruit, and the olive support the reproductive system. Adam and Eve ate from the fig tree. When they discovered they were naked, they felt ashamed. Notice the first shame is tied to the sexual organs.

How might you rise above shame?